Lean and green diet cookbook

Delicious green recipes to burn fat and boost your health

Lisa Reims

Table of contents

Pesto Zucchini Noodles

Time: 30 minutes

Serve: 4

Ingredients:

- 4 zucchini, spiralized
- 1 tbsp avocado oil
- 2 garlic cloves, chopped
- 2/3 cup olive oil
- 1/3 cup parmesan cheese, grated
- 2 cups fresh basil
- 1/3 cup almonds
- 1/8 tsp black pepper
- ¾ tsp sea salt

Instructions:

1. Add zucchini noodles into a colander and sprinkle with ¼ teaspoon of salt. Cover and let sit for 30 minutes. Drain zucchini noodles well and pat dry.

2. Preheat the oven to 400 F.

3. Place almonds on a parchment-lined baking sheet and bake for 6-8 minutes. Transfer toasted

almonds into the food processor and process until coarse.

4. Add olive oil, cheese, basil, garlic, pepper, and remaining salt in a food processor with almonds and process until pesto texture.

5. Heat the avocado-oil in a pan over medium to high heat. Add zucchini noodles and cook for 4-5 minutes.

6. Pour pesto over zucchini noodles, mix well and cook for 1 minute.

7. Serve immediately with baked salmon.

Nutrition: Calories 525 Fat 47.4 g Carbs 9.3 g Sugar 3.8 g Protein 16.6 g Cholesterol 30 mg

Baked Cod & Vegetables

Time: 30 minutes

Serve: 4

Ingredients:

- 1 lb cod fillets
- 8 oz asparagus, chopped
- 3 cups broccoli, chopped
- ¼ cup parsley, minced
- ½ tsp lemon pepper seasoning
- ½ tsp paprika
- ¼ cup olive oil
- ¼ cup lemon juice
- 1 tsp salt

Instructions:

Preheat the oven to 410 F. Cover the pan with baking paper and

1. Set aside.

2. In a small bowl, mix lemon juice, paprika, olive oil, lemon pepper seasoning, and salt.

3. Place fish fillets in the middle of the parchment paper. Place broccoli and asparagus around the fish fillets.

4. Pour lemon juice mixture over the fish fillets and top with parsley.

5. Bake in preheated oven for 13-15 minutes.

Nutrition: Calories 240 Fat 14.1 g Carbs 7.6 g Sugar 2.6 g Protein 23.7 g Cholesterol 56 mg

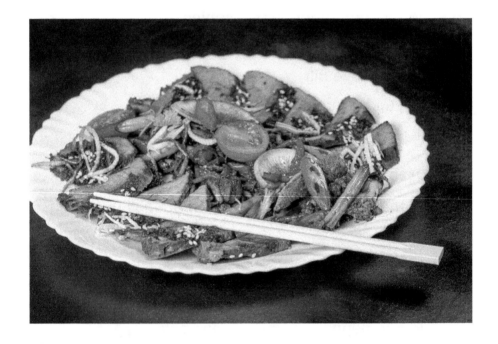

Parmesan Zucchini

Time: 30 minutes

Serve: 4

Ingredients:

- 4 zucchini, quartered lengthwise
- 2 tbsp fresh parsley, chopped
- 2 tbsp olive oil
- ¼ tsp garlic powder
- ½ tsp dried basil
- ½ tsp dried oregano
- ½ tsp dried thyme
- ½ cup parmesan cheese, grated
- Pepper
- Salt

Instructions:

1.Preheat the oven to 355 F. Line baking sheet with parchment paper and set aside.

2.In a small bowl, mix parmesan cheese, garlic powder, basil, oregano, thyme, pepper, and salt.

3.Arrange zucchini onto the prepared baking sheet and drizzle with oil and sprinkle with parmesan cheese mixture.

4. Cook for 16 minutes in a preheated oven, then broil for 2 minutes or until lightly browned.

5.Garnish with parsley and serve immediately.

Nutrition: Calories 244 Fat 16.4 g Carbs 7 g Sugar 3.5 g Protein 14.5 g Cholesterol 30 mg

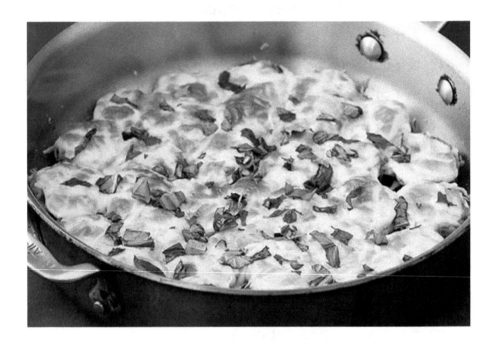

Chicken Zucchini Noodles

Time: 25 minutes

Serve: 2

Ingredients:

- 1 large zucchini, spiralized
- 1 chicken breast, skinless & boneless
- ½ tbsp jalapeno, minced
- 2 garlic cloves, minced
- ½ tsp ginger, minced
- ½ tbsp fish sauce
- 2 tbsp coconut cream
- ½ tbsp honey
- ½ lime juice
- 1 tbsp peanut butter
- 1 carrot, chopped
- 2 tbsp cashews, chopped
- ¼ cup fresh cilantro, chopped
- 1 tbsp olive oil
- Pepper
- Salt

Instructions:

Heat the olive oil in a pan.

1.Season chicken breast with pepper and salt. Add the chicken breast to the pan once the oil is hot and cook for 3-4 minutes on each side or until cooked.

2.Remove chicken breast from pan. Shred chicken breast with a fork and set aside.

3.In a small bowl, mix peanut butter, jalapeno, garlic, ginger, fish sauce, coconut cream, honey, and lime juice. Set aside.

4.In a large mixing bowl, combine spiralized zucchini, carrots, cashews, cilantro, and shredded chicken.

5.Pour peanut butter mixture over zucchini noodles and toss to combine.

Nutrition: Calories 353 Fat 21.1 g Carbs 20.5 g Sugar 10.8 g Protein 24.5 g Cholesterol 54 mg

Tomato Cucumber Avocado Salad

Time: 15 minutes

Serve: 4

Ingredients:

- 12 oz cherry tomatoes, cut in half
- 5 small cucumbers, chopped
- 3 small avocados, chopped
- ½ tsp ground black pepper
- 2 tbsp olive oil
- 2 tbsp fresh lemon juice
- ¼ cup fresh cilantro, chopped
- 1 tsp sea salt

Instructions:

1.Add cherry tomatoes, cucumbers, avocados, and cilantro into the large mixing bowl and mix well.

2.Mix olive oil, lemon juice, black pepper, and salt and pour over salad.

3.Toss well and serve immediately.

Nutrition: Calories 442 Fat 37.1 g Carbs 30.3 g Sugar 9.4 g Protein 6.2 g Cholesterol 0 mg

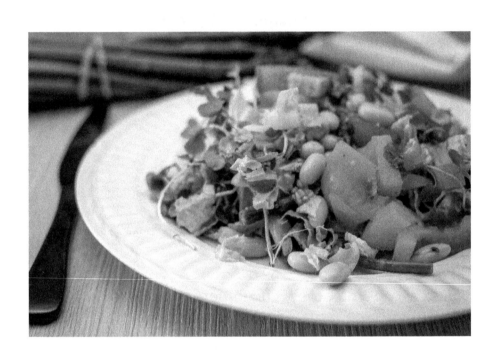

Creamy Cauliflower Soup

Time: 30 minutes

Serve: 6

Ingredients:

- 5 cups cauliflower rice
- 8 oz cheddar cheese, grated
- 2 cups unsweetened almond milk
- 2 cups vegetable stock
- 2 tbsp water
- 1 small onion, chopped
- 2 garlic cloves, minced
- 1 tbsp olive oil
- Pepper
- Salt

Instructions:

1. Heat olive-oil over medium heat in a big stockpot.

2. Add onion and garlic and cook for 1-2 minutes.

3. Add cauliflower rice and water. Cover and cook for 5-7 minutes.

3. Now add vegetable stock and almond milk and stir well. Bring to boil.

4. Turn heat to low and simmer for 5 minutes.

5.Turn off the heat. Slowly add cheddar cheese and stir until smooth.

6.Season soup with pepper and salt.

7.Stir well and serve hot.

Nutrition: Calories 214 Fat 16.5 g Carbs 7.3 g Sugar 3 g Protein 11.6 g Cholesterol 40 mg

Taco Zucchini Boats

Time: 70 minutes

Serve: 4

Ingredients:

- 4 medium zucchinis, cut in half lengthwise
- ¼ cup fresh cilantro, chopped
- ½ cup cheddar cheese, shredded
- ¼ cup of water
- 4 oz tomato sauce
- 2 tbsp bell pepper, mined
- ½ small onion, minced
- ½ tsp oregano
- 1 tsp paprika
- 1 tsp chili powder
- 1 tsp cumin
- 1 tsp garlic powder
- 1 lb lean ground turkey
- ½ cup of salsa
- 1 tsp kosher salt

Instructions:

1. Preheat the oven to 400 F.

2. Add ¼ cup of salsa to the bottom of the baking dish.

3.Using a spoon, hollow out the center of the zucchini halves.

4.Chop the scooped-out flesh of zucchini and set aside ¾ of a cup of chopped flesh.

5.Add zucchini halves to the boiling water and cook for 1 minute. Remove zucchini halves from water.

6.Add ground turkey in a large pan and cook until meat is no longer pink. Add spices and mix well.

7.Add reserved zucchini flesh, water, tomato sauce, bell pepper, and onion. Stir well and cover, simmer over low heat for 20 minutes.

8.Stuff zucchini boats with taco meat and top each with one tablespoon of shredded cheddar cheese.

9.Place zucchini boats in a baking dish. Cover the dish with paper and bake in a preheated oven

1. 35 minutes.

2. Top with remaining salsa and chopped cilantro.

Nutrition: Calories 297 Fat 13.7 g Carbs 17.2 g Sugar 9.3 g Protein 30.2 g Cholesterol 96 mg

Healthy Broccoli Salad

Time: 25 minutes

Serve: 6

Ingredients:

- 3 cups broccoli, chopped
- 1 tbsp apple cider vinegar
- ½ cup Greek yogurt
- 2 tbsp sunflower seeds
- 3 bacon slices, cooked and chopped
- 1/3 cup onion, sliced
- ¼ tsp stevia

Instructions:

1. In a mixing bowl, mix broccoli, onion, and bacon.

2. In a small bowl, mix yogurt, vinegar, and stevia and pour over broccoli mixture. Stir to combine.

3. Sprinkle sunflower seeds on top of the salad.

4. Store salad in the refrigerator for 30 minutes.

Nutrition: Calories 90 Fat 4.9 g Carbs 5.4 g Sugar 2.5 g Protein 6.2 g Cholesterol 12 mg

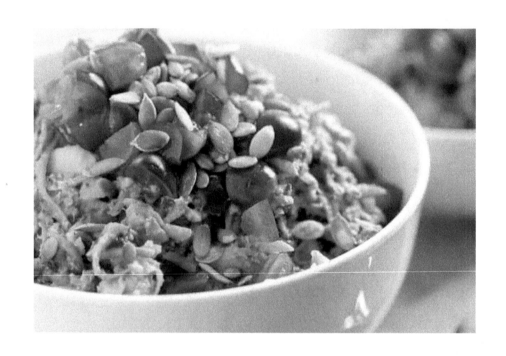

Delicious Zucchini Quiche

Time: 60 minutes

Serve: 8

Ingredients:

- 6 eggs
- 2 medium zucchini, shredded
- ½ tsp dried basil
- 2 garlic cloves, minced
- 1 tbsp dry onion, minced
- 2 tbsp parmesan cheese, grated
- 2 tbsp fresh parsley, chopped
- ½ cup olive oil
- 1 cup cheddar cheese, shredded
- ¼ cup coconut flour
- ¾ cup almond flour
- ½ tsp salt

Instructions:

1. Preheat the furnace to 355 F. Grease a 9-inch dish of pie and set aside.

2. Squeeze out excess liquid from zucchini.

3. Into the cup, add all ingredients and blend until well mixed. Pour into the prepared pie dish.

4. Bake in preheated oven for 47-63 minutes or until set.

5. Remove it from the oven and let it cool down completely.

Nutrition: Calories 288 Fat 26.3 g Carbs 5 g Sugar 1.6 g Protein 11 g Cholesterol 139 mg

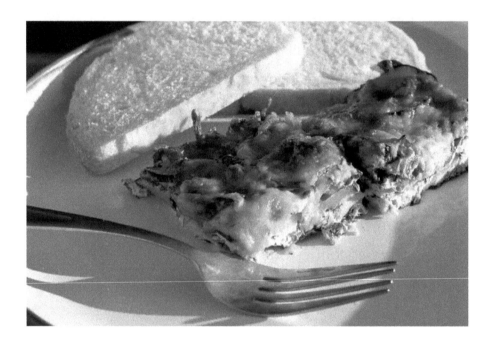

Turkey Spinach Egg Muffins

Time: 30 minutes

Serve: 3

Ingredients:

- 5 egg whites
- 2 eggs
- ¼ cup cheddar cheese, shredded
- ¼ cup spinach, chopped
- ¼ cup milk
- 3 lean breakfast turkey sausage
- Pepper
- Salt

Instructions:

1.Preheat the oven to 355 F. Grease muffin tray cups and set aside.

2.In a pan, brown the turkey sausage links over medium-high heat until the sausage is brown from all the sides.

3.Cut sausage into ½-inch pieces and set aside.

4.In a big bowl, whisk together eggs, egg whites, milk, pepper, and salt. Stir in spinach.

5.Pour egg mixture into the prepared muffin tray.

6.Divide sausage and cheese evenly between each muffin cup.

7.Bake in a preheated oven for 22 minutes or until muffins are set.

Nutrition: Calories 123 Fat 6.8 g Carbs 1.9 g Sugar 1.6 g Protein 13.3 g Cholesterol 123 mg

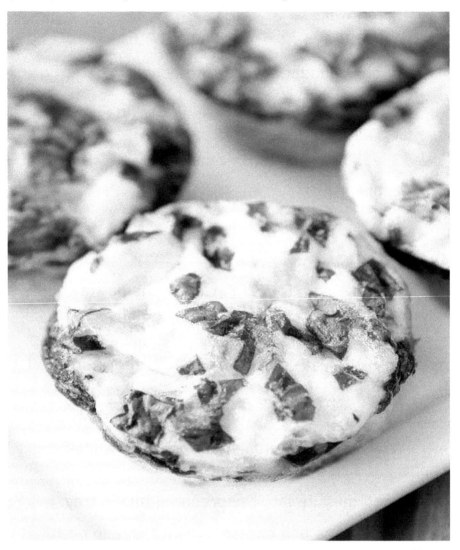

Chicken Casserole

Time: 40 minutes

Serve: 4

Ingredients:

- 1 lb cooked chicken, shredded
- ¼ cup Greek yogurt
- 1 cup cheddar cheese, shredded
- ½ cup of salsa
- 4 oz cream cheese, softened
- 4 cups cauliflower florets
- 1/8 tsp black pepper
- ½ tsp kosher salt

Instructions:

1.Add cauliflower florets into the microwave-safe dish and cook for 10 minutes or until tender.

2.Add cream cheese and microwave for 35 seconds more. Stir well.

3.Add chicken, yogurt, cheddar cheese, salsa, pepper, and salt, and stir everything well.

4.Preheat the oven to 375 F.

5.Bake in preheated oven for 20 minutes.

Nutrition: Calories 429 Fat 23 g Carbs 9.6 g Sugar 4.7 g Protein 45.4 g Cholesterol 149 mg

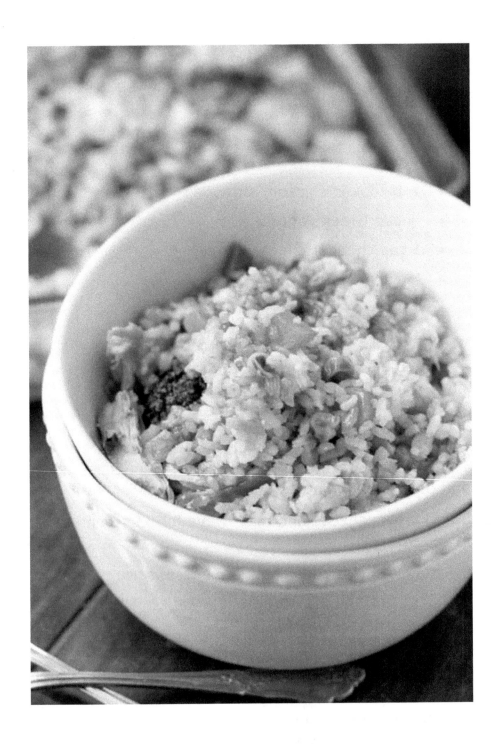

Shrimp Cucumber Salad

Time: 20 minutes

Serve: 4

Ingredients:

- 1 lb shrimp, cooked
- 1 bell pepper, sliced
- 2 green onions, sliced
- ½ cup fresh cilantro, chopped
- 2 cucumbers, sliced

For dressing:

- 2 tbsp fresh mint leaves, chopped
- 1 tsp sesame seeds
- ½ tsp red pepper flakes
- 1 tbsp olive oil
- ¼ cup rice wine vinegar
- ¼ cup lime juice
- 1 Serrano chili pepper, minced
- 3 garlic cloves, minced
- ½ tsp salt

Instructions:

1.In a little bowl, whisk together all dressing ingredients and set aside.

2.In a mixing bowl, mix shrimp, bell pepper, green onion, cilantro, and cucumbers.

3.Pour dressing over salad and toss well.

Nutrition: Calories 219 Fat 6.1 g Carbs 11.3 g Sugar 4.2 g Protein 27.7 g Cholesterol 239 mg

Asparagus & Shrimp Stir Fry

Time: 20 minutes

Serve: 4

Ingredients:

- 1 lb asparagus
- 1 lb shrimp
- 2 tbsp lemon juice
- 1 tbsp soy sauce
- 1 tsp ginger, minced
- 1 garlic clove, minced
- 1 tsp red pepper flakes
- ¼ cup olive oil
- Pepper and Salt

Instructions:

1.Heat 2 normal spoons of oil in a large pan over medium-high heat.

2.Add shrimp to the pan and season with red pepper flakes, pepper, salt, and cook for 5 minutes.

3.Remove shrimp from pan and set aside.

4.Add remaining oil in the same pan. Add garlic, ginger, and asparagus, stir frequently, and cook until asparagus is tender about 5 minutes.

5.Return shrimp to the pan. Add lemon-juice and soy-sauce and stir until well combined.

Nutrition: Calories 274 Fat 14.8 g Carbs 7.4 g Sugar 2.4 g Protein 28.8 g Cholesterol 239 mg

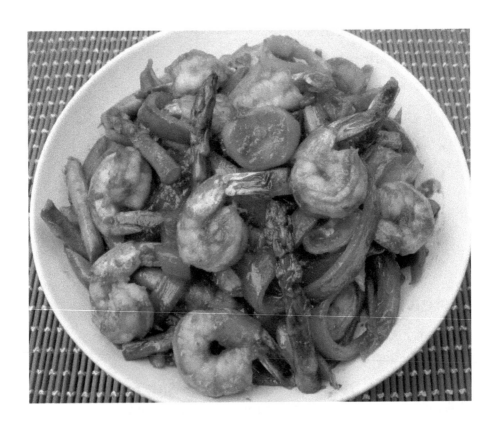

Turkey Burgers

Time: 30 minutes

Serve: 4

Ingredients:

- 1 lb lean ground turkey
- 2 green onions, sliced
- ¼ cup basil leaves, shredded
- 2 garlic cloves, minced
- 2 medium zucchini, shredded and squeeze out all the liquid
- ½ tsp black pepper
- ½ tsp sea salt

Instructions:

1.Heat grill to medium heat.

2.To the cup, add all the ingredients and combine until well blended.

3.Make four equal shapes of patties from the mixture.

4.Spray one piece of foil with cooking spray.

5.Place prepared patties on the foil and grill for 10 minutes. Turn patties to the other side and grill for 10 minutes more.

Nutrition: Calories 183 Fat 8.3 g Carbs 4.5 g Sugar 1.9 g Protein 23.8 g Cholesterol 81 mg

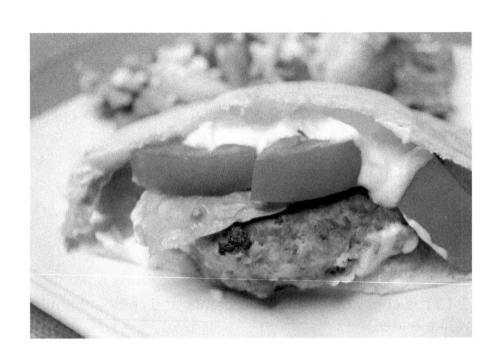

Broccoli Kale Salmon Burgers

Time: 30 minutes

Serve: 5

Ingredients:

- 2 eggs
- ½ cup onion, chopped
- ½ cup broccoli, chopped
- ½ cup kale, chopped
- ½ tsp garlic powder
- 2 tbsp lemon juice
- ½ cup almond flour
- 15 oz can salmon, drained and bones removed
- ½ tsp salt

Instructions:

1. Line one plate with parchment paper and set aside.

2. Add all ingredients into the big bowl and mix until well combined.

3. Make five equal shapes of patties from the mixture and place them on a prepared plate.

4. Place plate in the refrigerator for 30 minutes.

5. Spray a big pan with cooking spray and heat over medium heat.

6. Once the pan is hot, then add patties and cook for 5-7 minutes per side.

Nutrition: Calories 221 Fat 12.6 g Carbs 5.2 g Sugar 1.4 g Protein 22.1 g Cholesterol 112 mg

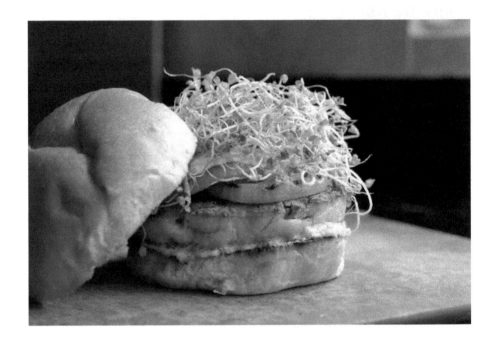

Pan Seared Cod

Time: 25 minutes

Serve: 4

Ingredients:

- 1 ¾ lbs cod fillets
- 1 tbsp ranch seasoning
- 4 tsp olive oil

Instructions:

1.Heat oil in a big pan over medium-high heat.

2.Season fish fillets with ranch seasoning.

3.Once the oil is hot, then place fish fillets in a pan and cook for 6-8 minutes on each side.

Nutrition: Calories 207 Fat 6.4 g Carbs 0 g Sugar 0 g Protein 35.4 g Cholesterol 97 mg

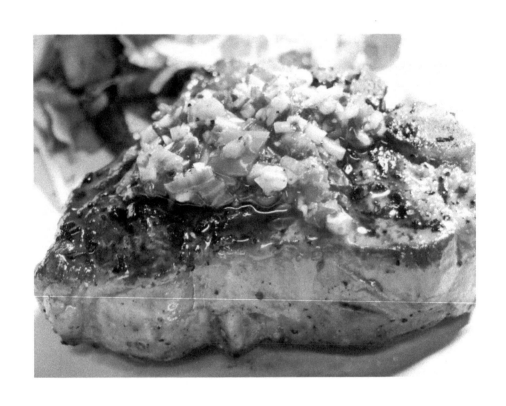

Quick Lemon Pepper Salmon

Time: 18 minutes

Serve: 4

Ingredients:

- 1 ½ lbs salmon fillets
- ½ tsp ground black pepper
- 1 tsp dried oregano
- 2 garlic cloves, minced
- ¼ cup olive oil
- 1 lemon juice
- 1 tsp sea salt

Instructions:

1.In a big bowl, mix lemon-juice, olive-oil, garlic, oregano, black pepper, and salt.

2.Add fish fillets in the bowl and coat well with the marinade, and place in the refrigerator for 15 minutes.

3.Preheat the grill.

4.Brush grill grates with oil.

5.Place marinated salmon fillets on hot grill and cook for 4 minutes, then turn salmon fillets to the other side and cook for 4 minutes more.

Nutrition: Calories 340 Fat 23.3 g Carbs 1.2 g Sugar 0.3 g Protein 33.3 g Cholesterol 75 mg

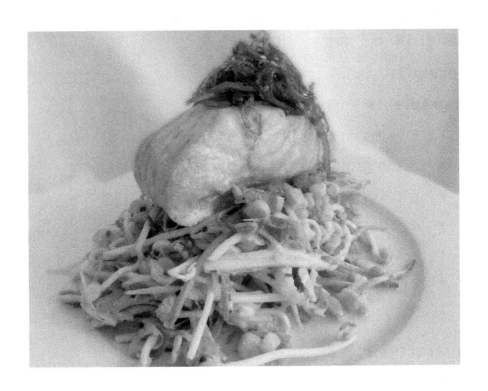

Healthy Salmon Salad

Time: 20 minutes

Serve: 2

Ingredients:

- 2 salmon fillets
- 2 tbsp olive oil
- ¼ cup onion, chopped
- 1 cucumber, peeled and sliced
- 1 avocado, diced
- 2 tomatoes, chopped
- 4 cups baby spinach
- Pepper and Salt

Instructions:

1. Heat the olive oil in a pan.

2. Season salmon fillets with pepper and salt. Place fish fillets in a pan and cook for 4-5 minutes.

3. Turn fish fillets and cook for 2-3 minutes more.

4. Divide remaining ingredients evenly between two bowls, then top with cooked fish fillet.

Nutrition: Calories 350 Fat 23.2 g Carbs 15.3 g Sugar 6.6 g Protein 25 g Cholesterol 18 mg

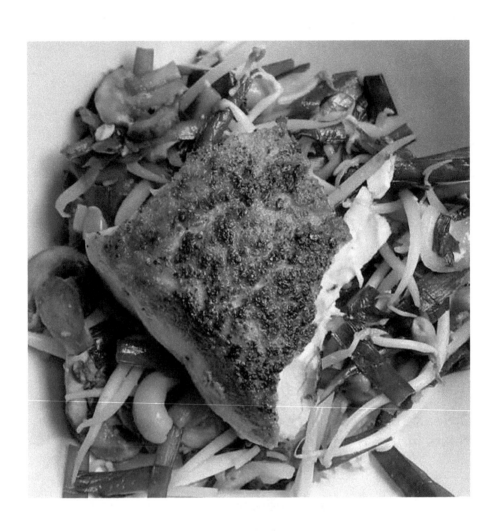

Pan Seared Tilapia

Time: 18 minutes

Serve: 2

Ingredients:

- 18 oz tilapia fillets
- ¼ tsp lemon pepper
- ½ tsp parsley flakes
- ¼ tsp garlic powder
- 1 tsp Cajun seasoning
- ½ tsp dried oregano
- 2 tbsp olive oil

Instructions:

1.Heat the olive oil in a pan.

2.Season fish fillets with lemon pepper, parsley flakes, garlic powder, Cajun seasoning, and oregano.

3.Place fish fillets in the pan and cook for 3-4 minutes on each side.

Nutrition: Calories 333 Fat 16.4 g Carbs 0.7 g Sugar 0.1 g Protein 47.6 g Cholesterol 124 mg

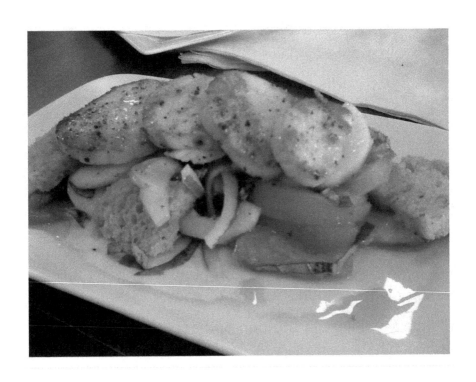

Creamy Broccoli Soup

Time: 35 minutes

Serve: 8

Ingredients:

- 20 oz frozen broccoli, thawed and chopped
- ¼ tsp nutmeg
- 4 cups vegetable broth
- 1 potato, peeled and chopped
- 2 garlic cloves, peeled and chopped
- 1 large onion, chopped
- 1 tbsp olive oil
- Pepper and Salt

Instructions:

1.Heat the olive oil in a pan.

2. Add the onion, garlic and sauté until the onion is tender.

3.Add potato, broccoli, and broth and bring to boil. Turn heat to low and simmer for 15 minutes or until vegetables are tender.

4.Using a blender, puree the soup until smooth. Season soup with nutmeg, pepper, and salt.

Nutrition: Calories 84 Fat 2.7 g Carbs 10.9 g Sugar 2.6 g Protein 5.1 g Cholesterol 0 mg

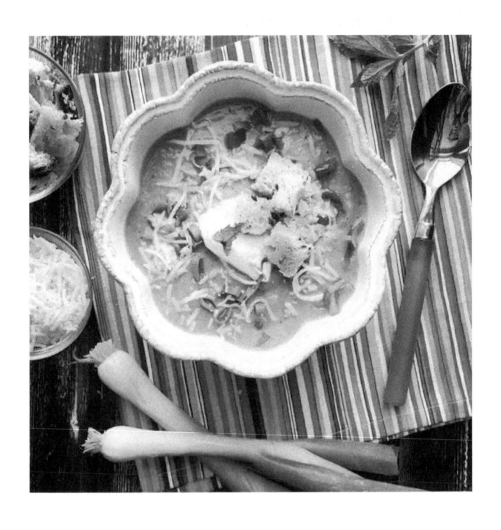

Tuna Muffins

Time: 35 minutes

Serve: 8

Ingredients:

- 2 eggs, lightly beaten
- 1 can tuna, flaked
- 1 tsp cayenne pepper
- 1/4 cup mayonnaise
- 1 celery stalk, chopped
- 1 1/2 cups cheddar cheese, shredded
- 1/4 cup sour cream
- Pepper and Salt

Instructions:

1.Preheat the oven to 355 F. Grease muffin tin and set aside.

2.Add all ingredients into the big bowl and mix until well combined, and pour into the prepared muffin tin.

3.Bake for 25 minutes.

Nutrition: Calories 185 Fat 14 g Carbs 2.6 g Sugar 0.7 g Protein 13 g Cholesterol 75 mg

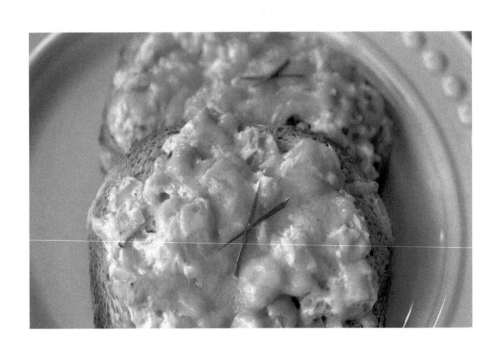

Chicken Cauliflower Rice

Time: 25 minutes

Serve: 4

Ingredients:

- 1 cauliflower head, chopped
- 2 cups cooked chicken, shredded
- 1 tsp olive oil
- 1 tsp garlic powder
- 1 tsp chili powder
- 1 tsp cumin
- 1/4 cup tomatoes, diced
- Salt

Instructions:

1.Add cauliflower into the food processor and process until you get rice size pieces.

2.Heat oil in a pan over high heat.

3.Add cauliflower rice and chicken in a pan and cook for 5-7 minutes.

4.Add garlic powder, chili powder, cumin, tomatoes, and salt. Stir well and cook for 7-10 minutes more.

Nutrition: Calories 140 Fat 3.6 g Carbs 5 g Sugar 2 g Protein 22 g Cholesterol 54 mg

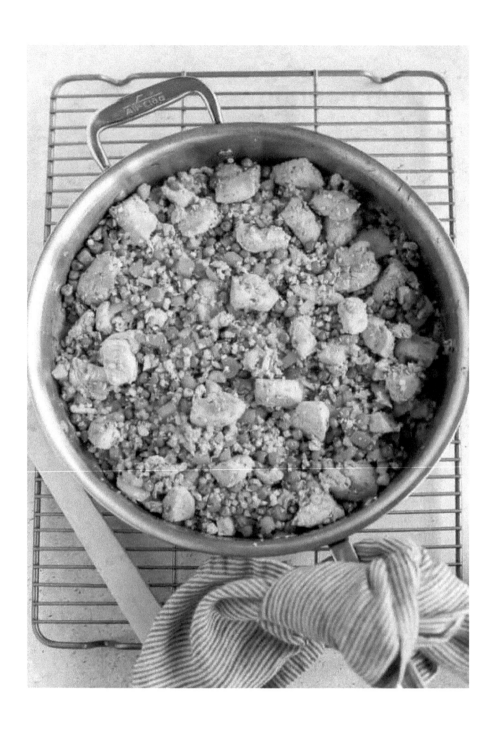

Easy Spinach Muffins

Time: 25 minutes

Serve: 12

Ingredients:

- 10 eggs
- 2 cups spinach, chopped
- 1/4 tsp garlic powder
- 1/4 tsp onion powder
- 1/2 tsp dried basil
- 1 1/2 cups parmesan cheese, grated
- Salt

Instructions:

1.Preheat the oven to 410 F. Grease muffin tin and set aside.

2.In a large bowl, whisk eggs with basil, garlic powder, onion powder, and salt.

3.Add cheese and spinach and stir well.

4.Pour egg-mixture into the prepared muffin tin and bake 15 minutes.

Nutrition: Calories 110 Fat 7 g Carbs 1 g Sugar 0.3 g Protein 9 g Cholesterol 165 mg

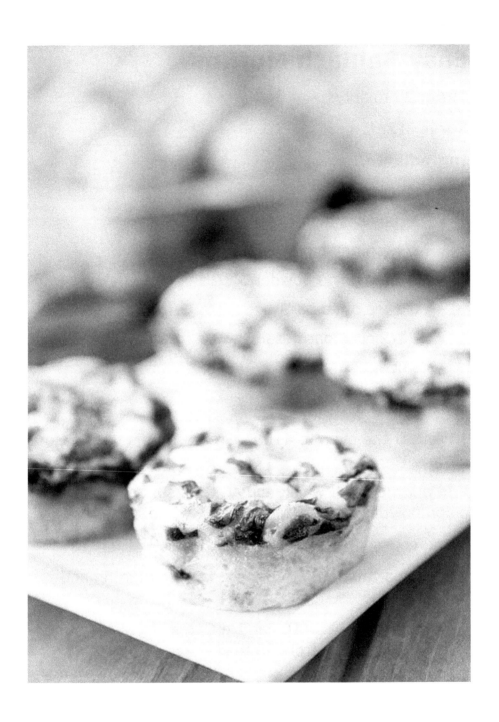

Healthy Cauliflower Grits

Time: 2 hours 10 minutes

Serve: 8

Ingredients:

- 6 cups cauliflower rice
- 1/4 tsp garlic powder
- 1 cup cream cheese
- 1/2 cup vegetable stock
- 1/4 tsp onion powder
- 1/2 tsp pepper
- 1 tsp salt

Instructions:

1. Add all the ingredients to the slow-cooker and blend well.

2. Cover and cook on low for 2 hours.

Nutrition: Calories 126 Fat 10 g Carbs 5 g Sugar 2 g Protein 4 g Cholesterol 31 mg

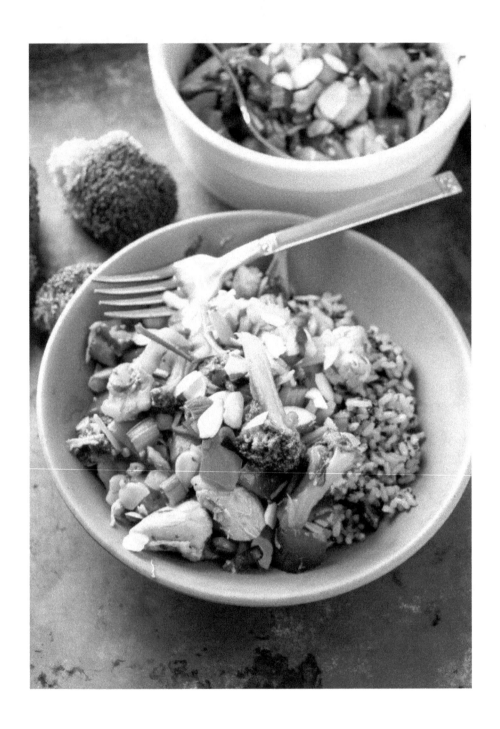

Spinach Tomato Frittata

Time: 30 minutes

Serve: 8

Ingredients:

- 12 eggs
- 2 cups baby spinach, shredded
- 1/4 cup sun-dried tomatoes, sliced
- 1/2 tsp dried basil
- 1/4 cup parmesan cheese, grated
- Pepper and Salt

Instructions:

1.Preheat the oven to 425 F. Grease oven-safe pan and set aside.

2.In a large bowl, whisk eggs with pepper and salt. Add remaining ingredients and stir to combine.

3.Pour egg-mixture into the prepared pan and bake for 20 minutes.

Nutrition: Calories 116 Fat 7 g Carbs 1 g Sugar 1 g Protein 10 g Cholesterol 250 mg

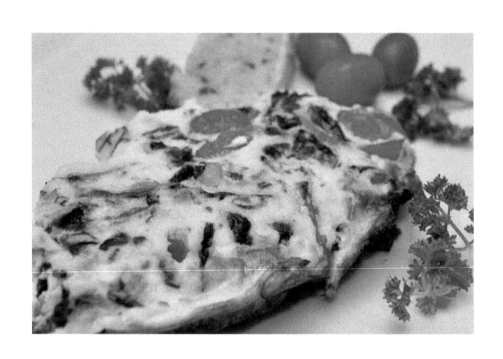

Tofu Scramble

Time: 17 minutes

Serve: 2

Ingredients:

- 1/2 block firm tofu, crumbled
- 1 cup spinach
- 1/4 cup zucchini, chopped
- 1 tbsp olive oil
- 1 tomato, chopped
- 1/4 tsp ground cumin
- 1 tbsp turmeric
- 1 tbsp coriander, chopped
- 1 tbsp chives, chopped
- Pepper and Salt

Instructions:

1.Heat the oil in a pan.

2.Add tomato, zucchini, and spinach and sauté for 2 minutes.

3.Add tofu, turmeric, cumin, pepper, and salt, and sauté for 5 minutes.

4.Garnish with chives and coriander.

Nutrition: Calories 102 Fat 8 g Carbs 5 g Sugar 2 g Protein 3 g Cholesterol 0 mg

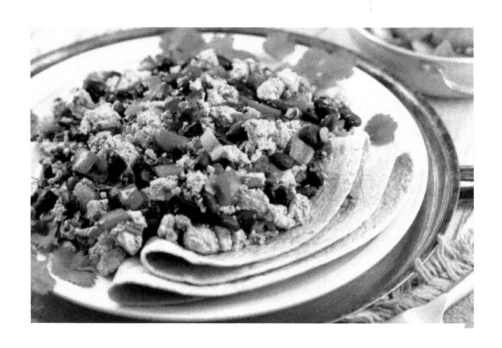

Shrimp & Zucchini

Time: 30 minutes

Serve: 4

Ingredients:

- 1 lb shrimp, peeled and deveined
- 1 zucchini, chopped
- 1 summer squash, chopped
- 2 tbsp olive oil
- 1/2 small onion, chopped
- 1/2 tsp paprika
- 1/2 tsp garlic powder
- 1/2 tsp onion powder
- Pepper and Salt

Instructions:

1.In a bowl, mix paprika, garlic powder, onion powder, pepper, and salt. Add shrimp and toss well.

2.Heat 1 normal spoon of oil in a pan over medium heat,

3.Add shrimp and cook for 2 minutes on each side or until shrimp turns pink.

4.Transfer shrimp on a plate.

5.Add remaining oil to a pan.

6.Add onion, summer squash, and zucchini, and cook for 6-8 minutes or until vegetables are softened.

7. Place the shrimp-back in the pan and cook for 1 minute.

Nutrition: Calories 215 Fat 9 g Carbs 6 g Sugar 2 g Protein 27 g Cholesterol 239 mg

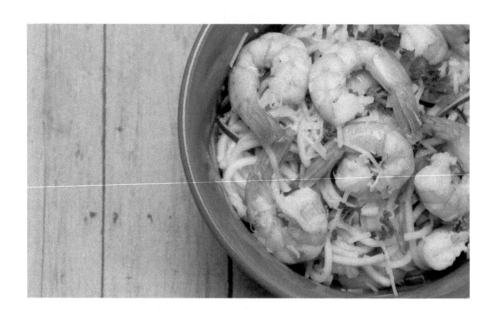

Baked Dijon Salmon

Time: 30 minutes

Serve: 5

Ingredients:

- 1 1/2 lbs salmon
- 1/4 cup Dijon mustard
- 1/4 cup fresh parsley, chopped
- 1 tbsp garlic, chopped
- 1 tbsp olive oil
- 1 tbsp fresh lemon juice
- Pepper and Salt

Instructions:

1.Preheat the oven to 385 F. Line baking sheet with parchment paper.

2.Arrange salmon fillets on a prepared baking sheet.

3.In a small bowl, mix garlic, oil, lemon juice, Dijon mustard, parsley, pepper, and salt.

4.Brush salmon top with garlic mixture.

5.Bake for 18-20 minutes.

Nutrition: Calories 217 Fat 11 g Carbs 2 g Sugar 0.2 g Protein 27 g Cholesterol 60 mg

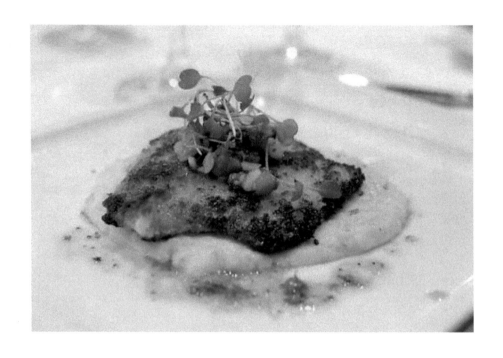

Cauliflower Spinach Rice

Time: 15 minutes

Serve: 4

Ingredients:

- 5 oz baby spinach
- 4 cups cauliflower rice
- 1 tsp garlic, minced
- 3 tbsp olive oil
- 1 fresh lime juice
- 1/4 cup vegetable broth
- 1/4 tsp chili powder
- Pepper and Salt

Instructions:

1.Heat the olive oil in a pan.

2.Add garlic and sauté for 30 seconds. Add cauliflower rice, chili powder, pepper, and salt and cook for 2 minutes.

3.Add broth and lime juice and stir well.

4.Add spinach and stir until spinach is wilted.

Nutrition: Calories 147 Fat 11 g Carbs 9 g Sugar 4 g Protein 5 g Cholesterol 23 mg

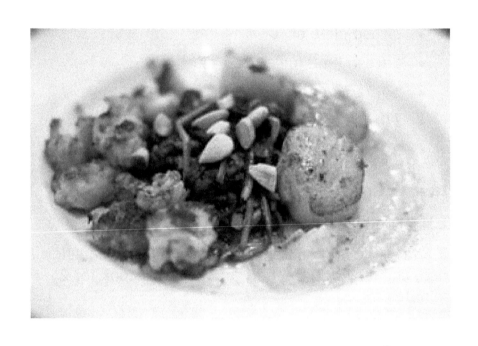

Cauliflower Broccoli Mash

Time: 22 minutes

Serve: 3

Ingredients:

- 1 lb cauliflower, cut into florets
- 2 cups broccoli, chopped
- 1 tsp garlic, minced
- 1 tsp dried rosemary
- 1/4 cup olive oil
- Salt

Instructions:

1.Add broccoli and cauliflower into the instant pot.

2.Pour enough water into the instant pot to cover broccoli and cauliflower.

3.Seal pot and cook on high-pressure for 12 minutes.

4.Once done, allow to release pressure naturally. Remove lid.

5.Drain broccoli and cauliflower and clean the instant pot.

6.Add oil into the instant pot and set the pot on sauté mode.

7.Add broccoli, cauliflower, rosemary, garlic, and salt, and cook for 10 minutes.

8.Mash the broccoli and cauliflower mixture using a masher until smooth.

Nutrition: Calories 205 Fat 17 g Carbs 12 g Sugar 5 g Protein 5 g Cholesterol 0 mg

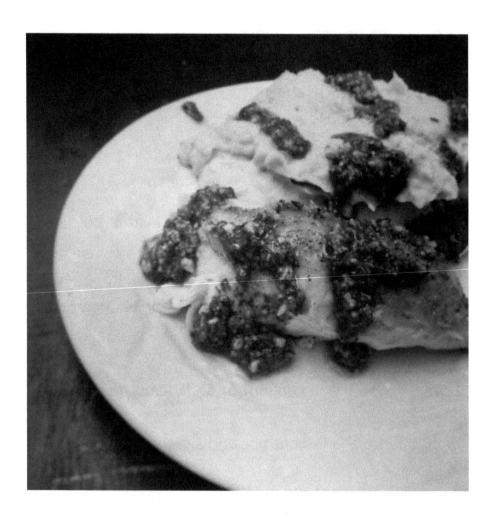

Italian Chicken Soup

Time: 35 minutes

Serve: 6

Ingredients:

- 1 lb chicken breasts, boneless and cut into chunks
- 1 1/2 cups salsa
- 1 tsp Italian seasoning
- 2 tbsp fresh parsley, chopped
- 3 cups chicken stock
- 8 oz cream cheese
- Pepper and Salt

Instructions:

1.Add all ingredients except cream cheese and parsley into the instant pot and stir well.

2.Seal pot and cook on high-pressure for 25 minutes.

3.Release pressure using quick release. Remove lid.

4.Remove chicken from pot and shred using a fork.

5.Return shredded chicken to the instant pot.

6.Add cream cheese and stir well and cook on sauté mode until cheese is melted.

Nutrition: Calories 300 Fat 19 g Carbs 5 g Sugar 2 g Protein 26 g Cholesterol 109 mg

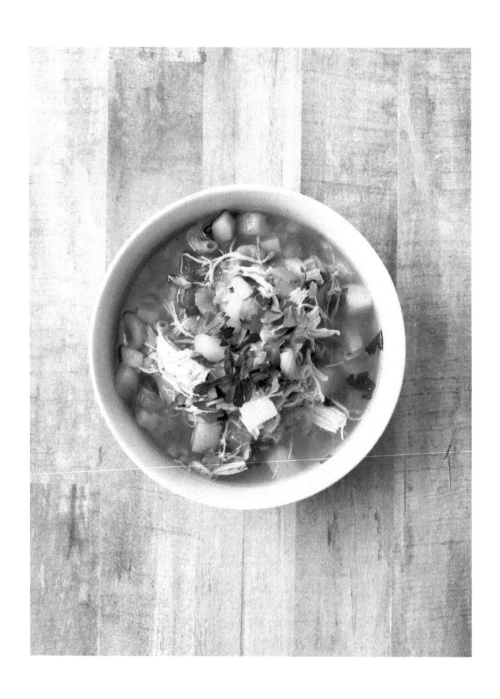

Tasty Tomatoes Soup

Time: 15 minutes

Serve: 2

Ingredients:

- 14 oz can fire-roasted tomatoes
- 1/2 tsp dried basil
- 1/2 cup heavy cream
- 1/2 cup parmesan cheese, grated
- 1 cup cheddar cheese, grated
- 1 1/2 cups vegetable stock
- 1/4 cup zucchini, grated
- 1/2 tsp dried oregano
- Pepper and Salt

Instructions:

1.Add tomatoes, stock, zucchini, oregano, basil, pepper, and salt into the instant pot and stir well.

2.Seal pot and cook on high-pressure for 5 minutes.

3.Release pressure using quick release. Remove lid.

4.Set pot on sauté mode. Add heavy cream, parmesan cheese, and cheddar cheese and stir well and cook until cheese is melted.

Nutrition: Calories 460 Fat 35 g Carbs 13 g Sugar 6 g Protein 24 g Cholesterol 117 mg

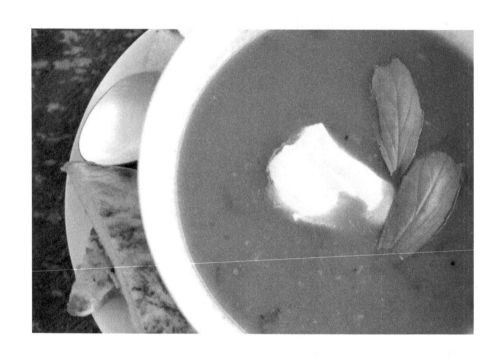

Cauliflower Spinach Soup

Time: 20 minutes

Serve: 2

Ingredients:

- 3 cups spinach, chopped
- 1 cup cauliflower, chopped
- 2 tbsp olive oil
- 3 cups vegetable broth
- 1/2 cup heavy cream
- 1 tsp garlic powder
- Pepper
- Salt

Instructions:

1.Add all ingredients except cream into the instant pot and stir well.

2.Seal pot and cook on high-pressure for 11 minutes.

3.Release pressure using quick release. Remove lid.

4.Stir in cream and blend soup using a blender until smooth.

Nutrition: Calories 310 Fat 27 g Carbs 7 g Sugar 3 g Protein 10 g Cholesterol 41 mg

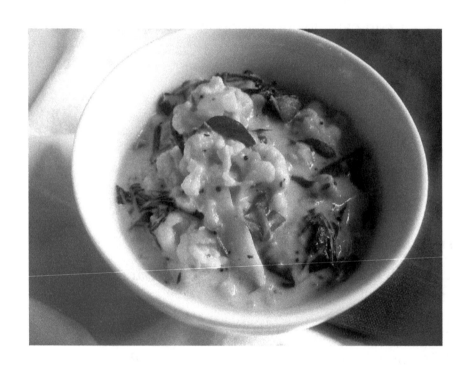

Delicious Chicken Salad

Time: 15 minutes

Serve: 4

Ingredients:

- 1 1/2 cups chicken breast, skinless, boneless, and cooked
- 2 tbsp onion, diced
- 1/4 cup olives, diced
- 1/4 cup roasted red peppers, diced
- 1/4 cup cucumbers, diced
- 1/4 cup celery, diced
- 1/4 cup feta cheese, crumbled
- 1/2 tsp onion powder
- 1/2 tbsp fresh lemon juice
- 1 tbsp fresh parsley, chopped
- 1 tbsp fresh dill, chopped
- 2 1/2 tbsp mayonnaise
- 1/4 cup Greek yogurt
- 1/4 tsp pepper
- 1/2 tsp salt

Instructions:

1.In a bowl, mix yogurt, onion powder, lemon juice, parsley, dill, mayonnaise, pepper, and salt.

2.Add chicken, onion, olives, red peppers, cucumbers, and feta cheese and stir well.

Nutrition: Calories 172 Fat 7.9 g Carbs 6.7 g Sugar 3.1 g Protein 18.1 g Cholesterol 52 mg

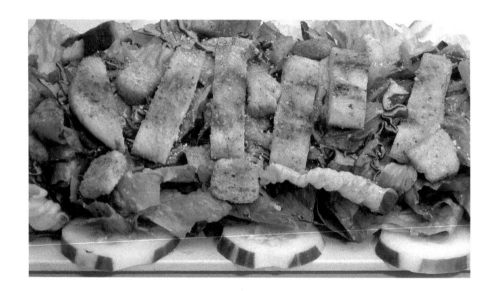

Baked Pesto Salmon

Time: 30 minutes

Serve: 5

Ingredients:

- 1 3/4 lbs salmon fillet
- 1/3 cup basil pesto
- 1/4 cup sun-dried to
- 1/4 cup olives, pitted and chopped
- 1 tbsp fresh dill, chopped
- 1/4 cup capers
- 1/3 cup artichoke hearts
- 1 tsp paprika
- 1/4 tsp

Instructions

1.Preheat the oven to 410 F. Cover the pan with parchment paper.

2.Arrange salmon fillet on a prepared baking sheet and season with paprika and salt.

3.Add remaining ingredients on top of salmon and spread evenly.

4.Bake for 20 minutes.

Nutrition: Calories 228 Fat 10.7 g Carbs 2.7 g Sugar 0.3 g Protein 31.6 g Cholesterol 70 mg

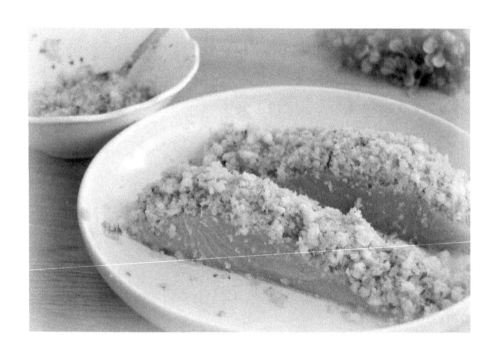

Easy Shrimp Salad

Time: 15 minutes

Serve: 6

Ingredients:

- 2 lbs shrimp, cooked
- 1/4 cup onion, minced
- 1/4 cup fresh dill, chopped
- 1/3 cup fresh chives, chopped
- 1/2 cup fresh celery, chopped
- 1/4 tsp cayenne pepper
- 1 tbsp fresh lemon juice
- 1 tbsp olive oil
- 1/4 cup mayonnaise
- 1/4 tsp pepper
- 1/4 tsp salt

Instructions:

1.In a big-bowl, add all ingredients except shrimp and mix well.

2.Add shrimp and toss well.

Nutrition: Calories 248 Fat 8.3 g Carbs 6.7 g Sugar 1.1 g Protein 35.2 g Cholesterol 321 mg

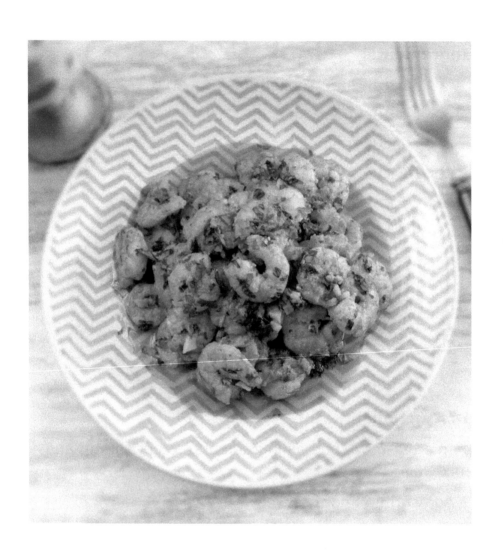

Simple Haddock Salad

Time: 15 minutes

Serve: 6

Ingredients:

- 1 lb haddock, cooked
- 1 tbsp green onion, chopped
- 1 tbsp olive oil
- 1 tsp garlic, minced
- Pepper and Salt

Instructions:

1.Cut cooked haddock into bite-size pieces and place on a plate.

2.Season with oil, pepper, and salt

3.Sprinkle garlic and green onion over haddock.

Nutrition: Calories 106 Fat 3 g Carbs 0.2 g Sugar 0 g Protein 18.4 g Cholesterol 56 mg

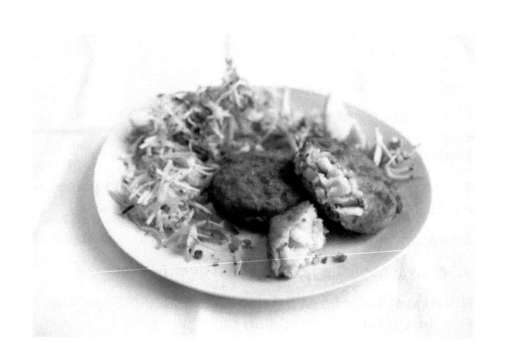

Baked White Fish Fillet

Time: 40 minutes

Serve: 1

Ingredients:

- 8 oz frozen white fish fillet
- 1 tbsp roasted red bell pepper, diced
- 1/2 tsp Italian seasoning
- 1 tbsp fresh parsley, chopped
- 1 1/2 tbsp olive oil
- 1 tbsp lemon juice

Instructions:

1.Preheat the oven to 410 F. Line baking sheet with foil.

2.Place a fish fillet on a baking sheet.

3.Drizzle oil and lemon juice over fish. Season with Italian seasoning.

4.Top with roasted bell pepper and parsley and bake for 30 minutes.

Nutrition: Calories 383 Fat 22.5 g Carbs 0.8 g Sugar 0.6 g Protein 46.5 g Cholesterol 2 mg

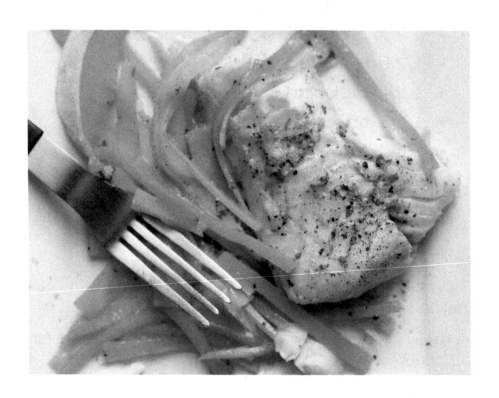

Air Fry Salmon

Time: 25 minutes

Serve: 4

Ingredients:

- 1 lbs salmon, cut into 4 pieces
- 1 tbsp olive oil
- 1/2 tbsp dried rosemary
- 1/4 tsp dried basil
- 1 tbsp dried chives
- Pepper and Salt

Instructions:

1.Place salmon-pieces skin side down into the air fryer basket.

2.In a small bowl, mix olive oil, basil, chives, and rosemary.

3.Brush salmon with oil mixture and air fry at 400 F for 15 minutes.

Nutrition: Calories 182 Fat 10.6 g Carbs 0.3 g Sugar 0 g Protein 22 g Cholesterol 50 mg

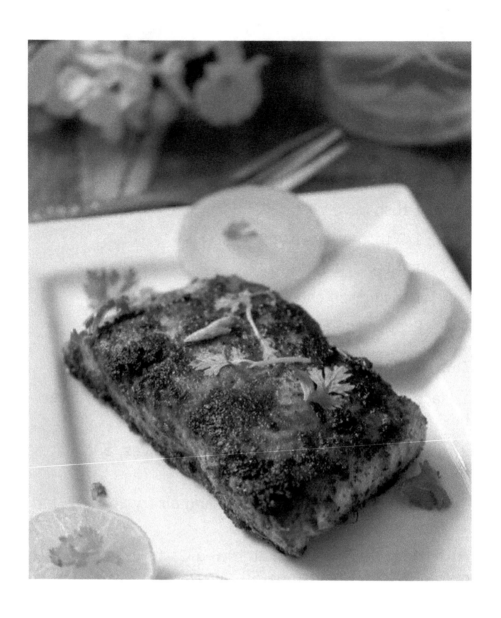

Baked Salmon Patties

Time: 30 minutes

Serve: 4

Ingredients:

- 2 eggs, lightly beaten
- 14 oz can salmon, drained and flaked with a fork
- 1 tbsp garlic, minced
- 1/4 cup almond flour
- 1/2 cup fresh parsley, chopped
- 1 tsp Dijon mustard
- 1/4 tsp pepper
- 1/2 tsp kosher salt

Instructions:

1. Preheat a 410 F microwave. Line a baking sheet and set it aside with parchment paper.

2.Add all ingredients into the bowl and mix until well combined.

3.Make small patties from the mixture and place on a prepared baking sheet.

4.Bake patties for 10 minutes.

5.Turn patties and bake for 10 minutes more.

Nutrition: Calories 216 Fat 11.8 g Carbs 3 g Sugar 0.5 g Protein 24.3 g Cholesterol 136 mg

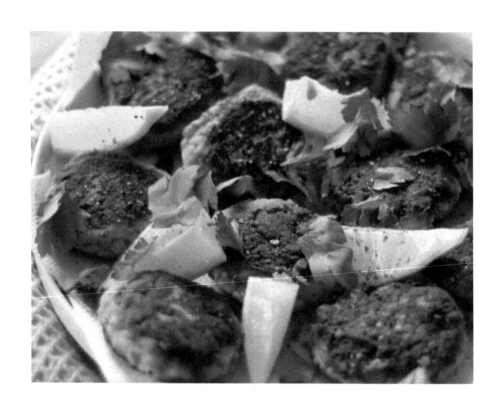

Peanut Butter Banana Sandwich

Prep Time: 2 minutes

Cook Time: 6 minutes

Serve: 1

Ingredients:

- 1 banana
- 1 tbsp. olive oil (or coconut oil)
- ½ tbsp. cinnamon
- 1 tbsp. peanut butter
- slices bread

Instructions:

1. On both slices of toast, smear the peanut butter.

2. Slice the banana into thin slices about 8 mm thick and spread them on just ONE toast slice.

3. Over them, add cinnamon.

4. Place all slices on each other's top.

5. For 2-3 minutes, apply oil to the pan and cook both faces until crispy and brown and yummy and delicious, and boom! Now, back to bed.

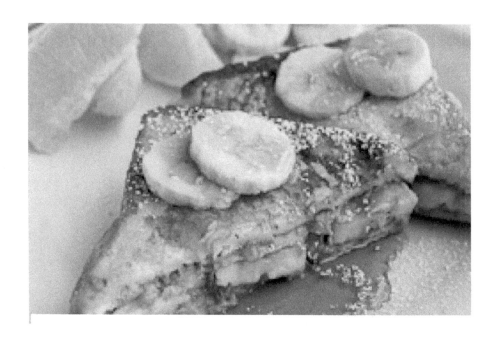

Tuna Pate

Prep Time: 15 min

Cook Time: 45 min

Serve: 6

Ingredients:

- 1/4 teaspoon pepper
- 1/4 teaspoon salt
- Grated rind of half an orange
- 2 tablespoons fresh parsley
- 1 can (6 ounces) tuna, drained
- 1 package (8 ounces) cream cheese, softened
- 1 can (4 ounces) mushrooms, drained
- 1/2 teaspoon orange extract
- 1 tablespoon Splendor
- 1/2 medium onion, chopped
- 2 cloves garlic, crushed
- 2 tablespoons butter

Instruction:

1. Melt the butter and stir-fry the onion and garlic, and mushrooms in a thin, heavy skillet over low heat until the onion is floppy. Connect the orange and Splendor extract and blend well.

2. With the S blade in, put the tuna, cream cheese, orange rind, parsley, salt, and pepper in a food mixer.

Pulse for mixing. Add the sautéed mixture, and pulse until well combined and smooth.

3. Cool and spoon into a mixing dish. Serve with (for carb-eaters) pepper strips, cucumber rounds, celery sticks, and crackers.

Nutrition: 3 g. carb. | 1 g. fib. for a total of 2 g. of usable carbs and 11 grams of protein.

Arugula Lentil Salad

Prep Time: 5 minutes

Cook Time: 7 minutes

Serve: 2

Ingredients:

- 1-2 tbsp. balsamic vinegar
- ¾ cups cashews (¾ cups = 100 g)
- 1 handful arugula/rocket (1 handful = 100 g)
- 1 cup brown lentils, cooked (1 cup = 1 / 15oz. / 400 g)
- slices bread (whole wheat)
- 5-6 sun-dried tomatoes in oil
- 1 chili / jalapeño
- tbsp. olive oil
- 1 onion
- salt and pepper to taste
- Optional
- 1 tbsp. honey
- 1 small handful of raisins

Instructions:

1. To optimize the scent, toast the cashews in a pan over low heat for about three to four minutes. Then dump them into a pot of salad.

2.Dice and fry the onion in one-third of the olive oil over low heat for around 3 minutes.

3.In the meantime, cut your chili / jalapeño and dried tomatoes. In the grill, add them and fry for the next 1-2 minutes.

4.Slice the bread into large croutons.

5.Shift the mixture of onions into a large container. Now add the remaaining oil to the pan and cook the sliced bread until it's crispy with salt and pepper seasoning.

6.Now clean the arugula and put it in the bowl.

7.Bring in the lentils, too, and blend everything over. Using salt, pepper, and balsamic vinegar to season. With the croutons, eat.

Tomato Avocado Toast

Prep Time: 5 min

Cook Time: 5 min

Serve: 1

Ingredients:

- 1 slice bread (ideally whole grain)
- ½ medium avocado (½ avocado = about 50g)
- 1 tbsp. lemon juice
- 1 tbsp. olive oil
- salt and pepper to taste
- cherry tomatoes

Instructions:

1.Split in half your cherry tomatoes.

2.Dump them in a pan and let them cook until tender (about 5 minutes) with olive oil.

3.In the meantime, mash and add some lemon with your avocado. Put it all together now, and season with salt and pepper.

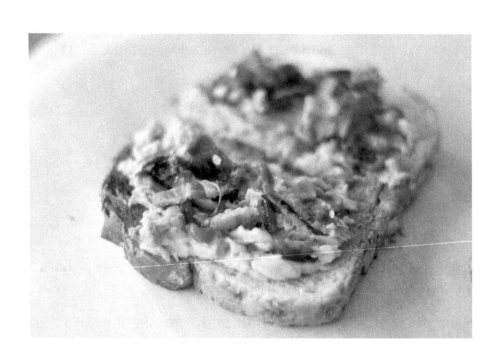

Classic Tofu Salad

Prep Time: 5 minutes

Cook Time: 15 minutes

Serve: 2

Ingredients:

- 1 small tin pineapple (small tin = 8 oz. = 225g = ¼)
- 1 handful spinach
- ½ bunch radishes
- ½ medium cucumber
- 1 cup bean sprouts
- 14 oz. firm tofu (ideally get fresh tofu from the supermarket)

For the dressing

- tbsp. olive oil
- salt and pepper to taste
- 1 small handful of peanuts
- ½ chili pepper (e.g., jalapeño)
- ½ lime (juiced; lemon also works)
- 1 tbsp. sriracha (or equivalent)
- 1 tbsp. maple syrup

Instructions:

1.Squeeze out some of the tofu block's excess moisture, split it (about one square centimeter) into tiny cubes, heat some oil in a pan over low to medium heat, and add it to your tofu. Fry until golden brown for approximately 15 minutes. Challenge for multitasking: make sure that you stir every once in a while (and put some salt). When preparing the rest of the salad, you should do it, get it on!

2.Next step: rinse the vegetables!

3.Chop the radishes.

4.Lengthwise, slice the cucumber in half, scrape the seeds with a big spoon, and cut what's left.

5.Also, cut the pineapple into smaller pieces.

6.Put all together with the bean sprouts and spinach into a dish.

Now to the dressing

1.Put the sugar, the olive oil, the sriracha, the lime juice, the salt, and the pepper together and toss in the salad

2.Get the pieces of tofu and put them in a separate bowl. Mix them to every

3.Serving of salad. (They'll get mushy easily if you put them straight into the salad).

4.Cut the chili and slightly crush or chop the peanuts for garnish as well. When served, dust them over the salad.

Two Ingredient Peanut Butter

Prep Time: 3 min

Cook Time: None

Serve: 8

Ingredients:

- 2 tbsp. olive oil
- 1 tbsp. maple syrup
- 1¼ cup peanuts

Instructions:

1.In a blender/food processor, add chunks of peanuts and oil (add maple syrup if desired).

2.Mix more for smooth texture, less for a crunchy blend.

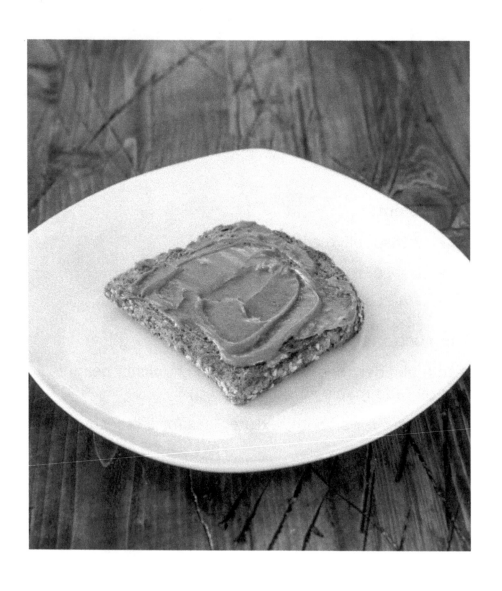

Avocado Toast with Cottage Cheese

Prep Time: 5 minutes

Cook Time: None

Serve: 1

Ingredients:

- 1 green onion
- 2 tbsp. cottage cheese
- 1 tbsp. lemon
- ½ medium avocado
- 1 slice bread (ideally whole grain)
- salt and pepper to taste

Instructions:

1.Mash the avocado; add the lemon and some salt.

2.On the toast, put a layer of cottage cheese.

3.Garnish with fresh pepper and sliced green onio.

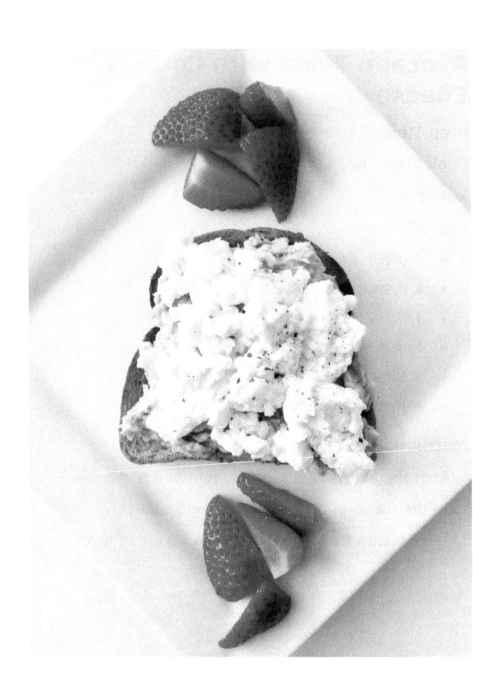

Creamy Corn Soup

Prep Time: 5 minutes

Cook Time: 15 minutes

Serve: 3

Ingredients:

- 1 pinch pepper (preferably freshly ground black pepper)
- 1 pinch salt
- 2 handfuls cilantro/coriander, fresh
- 2 tbsp. olive oil
- 2 cups vegetable broth (2 cups = ½ liter)
- 1 thumb ginger, fresh (or 1 tbsp. ground ginger)
- 2 cloves garlic
- 1 red pepper *
- 2 onion
- cans sweet corn (ca. 14oz. or 350-400g cans)

Optional and highly recommended:

- 1 tbsp. lemon juice (as an extra twist before serving)
- 2 stalks lemongrass (or 1 tbsp. ground lemongrass)

Instructions:

1.Heat the oven to a temperature of 430 ° F/220 ° C.

2.Flush the sweet corn in a different bowl, but save the water from the can!

3.To the baking tray, add 1/3 of the corn (without the water). Sprinkle with salt, pepper, and oil. Put it on for about 10 minutes in the oven. Stir periodically to make sure the maize is not burning.

4.Meanwhile, heat the remaining spoon of oil in a pan over medium heat.

5.Chop and sauté the onion (slowly fry it).

6.Peel the fresh ginger and chop it and transfer it to the onion. (Keep off a moment if dried ginger is used). For a moment, stir.

7.The garlic is sliced and added to the onion. Stir for around 30-60 seconds when the heat is low.

8.Now's the time to apply that to the mix and swirl for around 30-60 seconds if you're using freshly grated ginger (and optional: ground lemongrass).

9.Put the other 2 cans of corn and the liquid you set aside earlier (with the water / moist / broth from the can). The vegetable broth is also added and brought to a boil.

10.Make tiny slits in the lemongrass and apply them to the soup if you're using fresh lemongrass. Or, to slap the lemongrass a few times, use a wooden spoon. Later, as a whole, you can pull them out, so make sure that they remain in one piece.

11.Let the soup-boil on medium heat for around 10 minutes.

12.Regularly check on your oven-roasted corn. Meanwhile, cut the cilantro and slice the red pepper into small bits. If you don't want it hot, you want the red pepper first.

13.When the roasted corn is done (superbly golden, piping hot, popping here and there), put in the red pepper and coriander together to a cup. Just blend it well.

14.Remove the soup from the heat after ten minutes of boiling and mix it (a hand blender is ideal) until it's (kind of) smooth.

15.Serve the soup with the corn-coriander-red pepper mix in a teaspoon (or two!) of it.

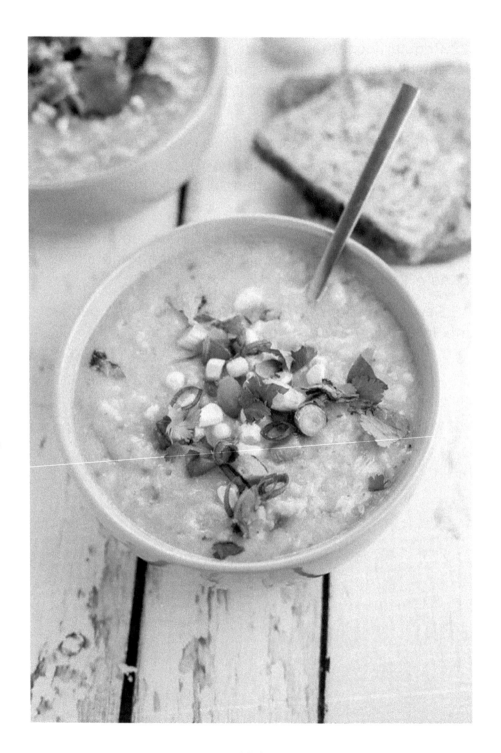

Egg on Avocado Toast

Prep Time: 3 minutes

Cook Time: 5 minutes

Serve: 1

Ingredients:

- slice bread
- salt and pepper to taste
- 1 tbsp. olive oil
- Sriracha
- 1 egg
- 1 tbsp. lemon
- ½ medium avocado

Instructions:

1.On medium-high heat, fry the egg and the toast in the pan with the olive oil.

2.In the meantime, mash the avocado, add salt and pepper, and put some lemon to the mixture.

3.Now add an egg to your toast.

4.Put a little bit of Sriracha and munches (or your favorite spicy sauce).

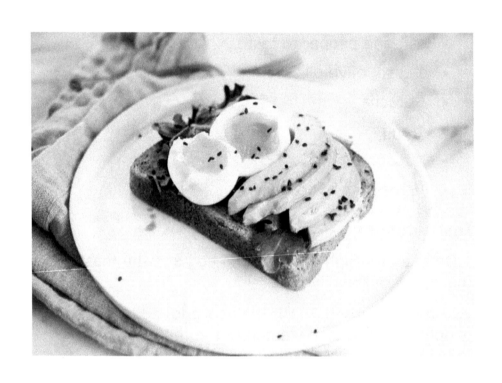

Moroccan Couscous Salad

Prep Time: 30 min

Cook Time: None

Serve: 6

Ingredients:

- 2 tbsp. olive oil
- fig, fresh (don't worry if you can't find one)
- ½ orange's zest
- orange
- 1 medium zucchini
- 1 pomegranate
- 1 tbsp. ginger powder (fresh is fine too. Chop it finely.)
- tbsp. cumin
- 1 tbsp. paprika powder
- 1 bell pepper, red
- ½ cup parsley, fresh
- 1 tbsp. salt
- salt and pepper to taste
- 1 cup of water
- ¼ cup raisins
- 1 cup instant couscous
- Optional
- bunch radish (thinly sliced)

Instructions:

1.Boil water in a wide serving bowl and apply it to the couscous.

2.Cover a tea towel or lid with the couscous and leave for 5 minutes.

3.Gently loosen the couscous with a fork and add the cumin, ginger, olive oil, and paprika powder. You want it dry and cool, no big clumps.

4.Wash the cherry, rub the zest.

5.Peel and chop the orange and, along with the zest, add it to the salad.

6.Deseed and apply the seeds to the pomegranate.

7.Finely cut the zucchini and thinly slice the red pepper. To the salad, add them.

8.Cut it upp and add it to the salad if you've managed to find a fig.

9.Clean the parsley and any other optional herbs, chop them, and then return them to the salad again.

10. Give a decent toss to it. It's that easy!

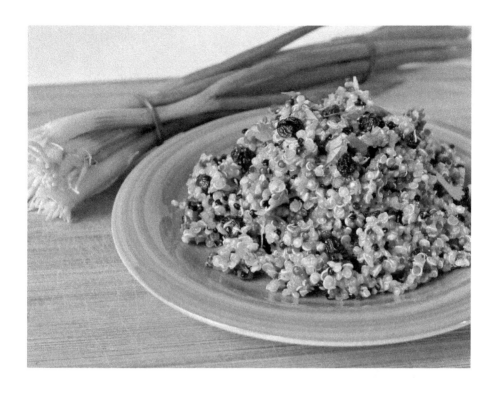